T0144722

Modified Citrus Pectin (MCP)

A Super Nutraceutical

Nan Kathryn Fuchs, Ph.D.

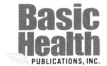

Basic Health PUBLICATIONS, INC.

Illustrations: Dorena Rode
Series Cover Designer: Mike Stromberg
Editor: Carol Rosenberg
Typesetter: Gary A. Rosenberg

Basic Health Guides are published by
Basic Health Publications, Inc.
www.basichealthpub.com

Contents

"Modified citrus pectin is a natural substance, it's non-toxic and it has been shown to slow down the progression of prostate cancer. I recommend MCP selectively to patients who have a high risk of recurrence of prostate cancer after any primary treatment. I also recommend MCP for those who have shown a slow, persistent rise of PSA levels that is consistent with established prostate cancer recurrence."

—Stephen Strum, M.D., Prostate Oncologist
Author, *A Primer on Prostate Cancer:
The Empowered Patient's Guide*

Introduction

Our most valuable medicines have their origins in plants. From the Brazilian shrub *Cephaelis ipecacuanha* that yields ipecac, a remedy for amoebic dysentery, to the bark of the Peruvian chinchona tree that gave us quinine, plants have helped us heal for centuries. Before the era of pharmaceutical drugs, plants and plant extracts were given for every complaint from minor ailments to major diseases. Through trial and error—and through careful observation—ancient doctors learned the properties of each plant. Out of their observations came the first human clinical trials.

Research has become more sophisticated since then, and we now have the ability to extract particular plant molecules. But today's medicine, both traditional and complementary, has its roots in ancient times with plants. The pattern today is to discover the active ingredients in plants and turn them into pharmaceutical drugs as fast as possible. Pharmaceutical companies then charge high sums of money for these synthetic drugs, making it impossible for many people to afford them. What's more, many of these drugs have side effects, limiting their long-term usefulness.

At the same time that pharmaceutical companies look for the perfect drug, independent researchers with far fewer funds are studying plant materials looking for natural, less-toxic solutions to our health problems. Pharmaceutical companies pour money into researching and promoting drugs they can patent. Since few natural products can be patented, there is less research on natural products. One exception is modified citrus pectin (MCP), a super nutraceutical with impressive research behind it.

MCP starts out as ordinary pectin and is transformed into a natural product with enhanced capabilities. When it has been properly modified, MCP can keep cancer cells from attaching to the walls or blood vessels (their source of nutrients) or to one another. This keeps them from forming into tumors and from spreading to other sites. But cancer prevention and treatment are only two of its many applications. As recent clinical trials are showing, MCP has a significant role in reducing heart disease and removing toxins.

The discovery of MCP, and the MCP product found in studies to have the most optimal characteristics, is a fascinating story that has not been told before. It begins thirty years ago in Israel when scientists were studying the peel of oranges and grapefruits for any health benefits. And the final chapter has yet to be written.

Pectin is a common soluble fiber that's found in large quantities in apple skins and the rinds of citrus fruits. It's made from a long chain of sugar molecules. You may be familiar with using apple pectin in making jams and jellies. It gives them body and a smooth texture. Or you may have used a combination of kaolin clay and pectin to successfully stop diarrhea. As a bulking agent, pectin is also included in some preparations to reduce and eliminate constipation. But this simple fiber does much more. Because it is a soluble fiber, pectin also helps lower cholesterol, reducing your risk for heart disease. But because pectin's molecules are too large to be digested and absorbed into the bloodstream, its actions are limited to its activity in the digestive tract.

The value of pectin increased substantially when scientists modified its larger molecules into smaller, less complex ones. This new substance, called modified citrus pectin (or MCP), has smaller molecules that dissolve better in water than ordinary pectin's, increasing its absorption substantially. These smaller molecules are able to travel across the intestinal lining and through the bloodstream where it can interact with other cells in the blood or in tissues.

MCP is one of the most exciting nutraceuticals available today to improve the quality and length of your life. It does everything that pectin alone can do—and much more. Ordinary pectin is useful. Modified citrus pectin is an invaluable nutrient for everyone who wants protection against cancer, cancer progression, and heart disease. By preventing these two major age-associated illnesses, MCP is truly an anti-aging supplement.

It excels as an anticancer nutrient by stopping tumor growth and preventing primary tumors from spreading to other sites. This not only reduces the risk of getting cancer, but it also protects against recurring malignancy as well, even for those people with a genetic predisposition for this disease. MCP guards against heart disease by lowering cholesterol levels and reducing arteriosclerosis. It also removes an underlying cause of many chronic illnesses—heavy metal toxicity.

The preliminary research studying the effects of MCP on animals and humans is compelling, and the implications for future use of this nutrient are exciting. More research is underway, and the completed studies place MCP high on the list of cutting-edge nutraceuticals that are vital for health, longevity, and anti-aging.

1. How Pectin Can Improve Your Health

Many plants contain pectin, but this soluble fiber is found most abundantly in apples, oranges, lemons, and grapefruit. While pectin is most commonly used as a bulking agent to relieve constipation, a number of studies indicate that its usefulness as a soluble fiber can protect against colon cancer. A study published in the *Journal of the National Cancer Institute* in 1979, comparing various types of fiber, found that pectin was one of the most protective forms in preventing colon cancer in laboratory animals.

Apple pectin and citrus pectin are similar, but their actions are not identical. Citrus pectin has superior binding capabilities, while apple pectin works primarily as a bulking agent. Researchers are discovering that citrus pectin has an even greater number of health benefits than apple pectin.

Pectin Reduces Your Risk of Colon Cancer

The longer waste products remain in your intestines, the more likely they are to break down into cancer-promoting materials and the greater your risk becomes for getting colon cancer. In thirteen studies, there was a significant decrease in colon cancer rates when dietary fiber was increased. Fiber is like a broom that binds to potentially dangerous toxic wastes in the stool and sweeps them out of the body. Pectin is an ideal fiber for this job.

During normal fermentation in the colon, pectin forms a fatty acid called butyric acid. It is thought that the butyric acid and fiber in pectin both bind to potential mutagens—substances that can become malignant—enhancing pectin's binding capacities. By attaching them-

selves to toxins in solid wastes and removing them from the intestines, pectin helps prevent colon cancer. Perhaps this is one way "An
apple a day keeps the doctor away." Ordinary pectin has value
throughout the intestinal tract, but after it has been modified into a
product with smaller molecules, this new form has additional anticancer activities that far exceed those of pectin—even for colon cancer. These will be discussed later in more detail.

Pectin Lowers Cholesterol

A number of studies have shown that pectin lowers both total cholesterol and LDL, the harmful cholesterol that causes a buildup of
plaque in the arteries. But pectin's cholesterol-lowering activities are
limited by its inability to be absorbed into the bloodstream. High-vis-
cosity pectin may be thick enough to interfere with the body's
absorption of cholesterol through the intestinal walls, but it can't get
directly into the bloodstream. However, when less cholesterol is
absorbed in the intestines, one side effect is an additional reduction
of cholesterol in the bloodstream. To get directly into the bloodstream, pectin's molecules need to be modified. The end result is a
substance called modified citrus pectin.

2. What Is Modified Citrus Pectin (MCP)?

Modified citrus pectin is a form of pectin that has had some of its properties altered in one of several laboratory processes. These alterations, such as changing the size of its molecules to enable it to be better absorbed, give it enhanced capabilities. The seeds for today's high-quality modified citrus pectin were sown more than thirty years ago in Israel at a time when the oranges and grapefruits grown in that country were prized and known throughout Europe for their size and flavor. At that time, Israeli scientists were examining all aspects of these citrus fruits, and studying their properties.

Drs. Ruth and Leo Cohen were two of these scientists. Each of them held Ph.D.s in organic chemistry and each were pioneers in the citrus industry. Their specialty was the extraction and preservation of various components of citrus fruits. In addition, Dr. Leo Cohen's expertise was in the narrow field of citrus pectins.

One day, their inquisitive twelve-year-old neighbor, Isaac Eliaz, paid one of his frequent visits to the Cohen's. That particular afternoon still stands out vividly in his mind. Seemingly from out of nowhere, Dr. Ruth Cohen said to him, "Isaac, one day they will find out that there is a cure for cancer in the peel of the orange." It was a statement that could have been lost forever. But for some reason, that small boy never forgot it. Thirty years later, he had become a medical doctor practicing in the United States with a specialty in integrative medicine. His main interest was in finding the cancer-fighting properties in foods to help prevent and reverse cancers. As he found various substances with anticancer properties, he studied them and added them to his treatment protocols for his patients.

Perhaps living near scientists who were always talking about their research influenced him. Perhaps it was his natural curiosity. For whatever the reason, Dr. Eliaz found he was not interested in the many unsubstantiated claims he heard about various substances. He always looked to the science behind each of them. In 1995, he came upon the first paper by Dr. Kenneth J. Pienta who had conducted an animal study on the use of citrus pectin for the prevention of prostate cancer metastasis to the lungs. Prostate cancer cells frequently break off from the primary tumor and migrate to other areas, including the lungs. In this study, Dr. Pienta found that pectin prevented this spread of cancer from the prostate to the lungs. The results of this study were impressive, and Dr. Eliaz immediately recalled the conversation he had with his former neighbor decades before. Picking up the phone, he dialed the Cohen's old number in Israel. Remarkably, Dr. Ruth Cohen answered.

"Ruth . . . Do you remember what you told me so many years ago?" Isaac asked, excitedly. "You were right!" This marked the beginning of a dialogue between the two of them that would put Dr. Eliaz in touch with the premier international expert on citrus pectin, Prof. Pilnik, who lived in The Netherlands.

Although Prof. Pilnik was retired, he was still in touch with the best scientists in the world who were working in the field of pectins. Prof. Pilnik was so captivated by Dr. Eliaz's enthusiasm that he put him in touch with his colleagues so he could develop exactly the right preparation. The search had begun for a citrus pectin product with the precise molecular size and weight to be able to move from the intestines into the bloodstream. This was vital, because it had become clear to Dr. Eliaz after reading the studies on pectin and speaking with these scientists that pectin had an additional ability that could revolutionize the field of complementary medicine. If it could reach cancer cells, pectin could stop them from spreading or growing.

The production of the ideal form of modified citrus pectin (MCP) follows Dr. Eliaz's journey from the larger-molecule structure of citrus pectin to understanding the additional health benefits present in the smaller-molecule MCP. The more he read and spoke with researchers, the more applications there seemed to be for a modified pectin product. Like many discoveries, this one took place because a young doctor remembered what his neighbor had told him thirty years before. From that point, everything else fell into place. Clearly, the right people were in the right place at the right time.

As he studied MCP more closely, Dr. Eliaz began to understand that all forms of modified pectin were not alike. In order to have the beneficial properties he was seeking, citrus pectin needed to be modified in a very specific way. It had to be the precise molecular weight and have the proper structure. It took him years, with a great deal of help from knowledgeable scientists worldwide, to discover which preparation was the very best. There are patents that exist for products, and patents for the application of particular products. At present, Dr. Eliaz holds patents on the application of modified citrus pectin for cancer, atherosclerosis, and binding to toxins and heavy metals.

MCP's Weight and Structure

To understand MCP, we need to first look at its chemical structure. Pectin is a long-chain polysaccharide. This simply means that it is made up of a long string of sugar molecules. In fact, two-thirds of these molecules closely resemble the sugar galactose. Because pectin is primarily made up of sugars, it has a particular affinity to molecules that bind to sugars. In a little while, you'll understand just how important this is in the area of cancer prevention and treatment.

Pectin's properties are restricted because of its size. It cannot be broken down in the intestines and its molecules are too large to be absorbed into the bloodstream. While this makes it a valuable substance for intestinal conditions like constipation and the prevention of colon cancer, it limits most of its other possible effects. The smaller its molecules are—up to a point—the better pectin can be absorbed and the more applications it has. But before it can become a valuable nutritional supplement with increased health-enhancing properties, its very structure, along with the size and weight of its molecules, needs to be altered. The long chain of sugar molecules needs to be broken down into smaller ones, and its degree of esterification (which will be explained later) needs to be reduced. The result is the exciting new product we know as modified citrus pectin (MCP).

How Pectin Is Modified

When its larger molecules are broken down into smaller ones, MCP takes on a different molecular weight than ordinary citrus pectin. There are several ways this can be done. The best and most expensive method is an enzymatic process that chops pectin's long molecular chain into smaller, uniform pieces. The less expensive method is a process that uses sodium hydroxide (otherwise known as lye) along with an acid that breaks down pectin's molecules into smaller, non-uniform fragments. This second process, which consists of modifying the pH, typically cannot produce molecules smaller than 30,000 daltons. Studies indicate that pectin's molecules should be between 10,000 and 20,000 daltons for optimal absorption. This larger molecular size has not yet been evaluated for effectiveness in scientific studies.

The highest-quality modified citrus pectin is produced using an expensive enzymatic process that produces a product with molecules between 10,000 and 20,000 daltons all of uniform size. Presently, it is only found in a product called PectaSol®. The reason this MCP is highest in quality is that when pectin's molecules are of uniform size, more of them can get to the target areas. It takes less of a high-quality MCP to be effective than one of a lower quality that has molecules of different sizes. We won't know how other MCPs compare with Pecta-Sol until there are studies using each of them.

Pectin's Molecular Weight

The size of the molecules in pectins, expressed as molecular weight, determines where they can go and what they can do. The majority of the molecules in unmodified citrus pectins are between 50,000 and 150,000 daltons. These are the large molecules that are limited to traveling within the intestinal tract. Before pectin can be absorbed through the intestinal lining and get into the bloodstream, research shows that its molecules must be modified into smaller pieces that are between 10,000 and 20,000 daltons. This results in a modified citrus pectin with enhanced capabilities.

There is no standardization for MCPs, and the molecular weight of products on the market varies greatly from around 5,000 to 30,000 daltons. It might appear at first that the smaller the molecules, the better the product. But this doesn't seem to be the case. MCP with the smallest molecules—around 5,000 daltons—appears to break down quickly and may be too small for the immune system to recognize. Those, on the other hand, with a molecular weight of 30,000 daltons may be too large to be well absorbed. Without further research on MCPs with differing molecular weights, there's no way to know what their properties are.

We do know from cell culture studies that Dr. Eliaz conducted on pectins with varying molecular weights that all MCPs do not produce the same results.

He found that pectins with either smaller or larger molecules were less effective against cancer than those with a molecular weight of between 10,000 and 20,000 daltons. MCP with this molecular weight is small enough to be absorbed into the blood, small enough to circulate to other places, but not too small so that it gets broken down and eliminated by the body very quickly. Before we know the effectiveness—or limitations—of MCPs with molecular weights outside of this range, researchers will need to conduct extensive studies with them.

3. Cancer and the Role of Galectins

When cells are healthy, they regenerate, replacing themselves in an orderly, controlled way. As one cell becomes sick and dies, another is produced to replace it. Some cells, however, grow at an accelerated rate. As these cells pile up, they form tumors. When tumor cells look normal and are self-contained, the tumor is benign. It doesn't invade other tissues or travel through the bloodstream and attach itself to organs.

Cancer cells, on the other hand, are abnormal cells that either aren't sick enough to die and be replaced, or are somehow able to protect themselves from dying. In either case, these cells multiply into a tumor and can spread by invading healthy tissues. This process is called metastasis. Obviously, one way to stop the progression of malignant (cancerous) tumors is to stop metastasis. Most types of cancers can be stopped or prevented by destroying galectins—particularly one of them called galectin-3.

Recent research at Wayne State University, published in the *Journal of National Cancer Institute* (December 2002) suggests that galectin-3 is involved in the formation of new blood vessels, a process known as angiogenesis. Cancer cells are hungry cells that need a constant supply of the nutrients that they get from blood vessels. If there are no blood vessels near emerging tumors, the body will produce them. This university study found that MCP reduced tumor growth, angiogenesis, and metastasis in tumors containing galectin-3. So, in addition to stopping the progression of cancer and reversing it, MCP appears to have anti-angiogenetic properties.

What Are Galectins?

Galectins are proteins on the surface of cells that function like sticky hands by helping cells connect to one another. Galectins have a particular affinity for all sugars. Cells attach themselves to one another when galectins bind to galactose—a sugar molecule found on the surface of neighboring cells.

In addition to attaching cells to one another, galectins provide an important way for cells to communicate. Just as we can say "hello" or "stop" with our hands, galectins allow the different cells in a tissue to hold on to one another and relay messages about their cellular needs to neighboring cells.

Normal cells have a few galectins while cancerous cells have many. In fact, the more galectins there are on a cancer cell, the more dangerous and aggressive the cancer cell. When a cancer cell has numerous galectins, it can readily attach itself to other cells and eventually invade neighboring tissues. This explains why the more developed advanced cancers have the greatest number of galectins on their cells.

There are nearly a dozen different galectins, but at this time, galectin-3 has been more rigorously studied than the others, and it appears to play a key role in the development and spread of cancers.

What Does Galectin-3 Do?

Galectin-3 has three major roles in the progression of cancer:

1. It allows cancer cells to bind together and form groups of cancer cells so they can survive in the bloodstream and travel to other sites.

2. It allows groups of cancer cells that have broken away from a primary tumor to attach themselves to a new site, forming a new tumor. This process is called metastasis.

3. Cancer cells are hungry cells, and malignant tumors need blood vessels to supply them with nutrients. Galectin-3 interacts with blood vessels to stimulate new blood vessel growth (angiogenesis) if no blood supply exists near the tumor.

Galectin-3

Free
Cancer Cells

**Cancer cells form
tumors by binding via
galectin-3 molecules.**

The Role of MCP in Cancer

MCP binds to galectins, and by doing so, it prevents tumor forma-tion, the spread of cancer, and angiogenesis.

MCP Surrounds and Blocks Galectins

Tumors are created when the galectins on a cell attach themselves to other cells, forming clusters. As these clusters grow, they become tumors. MCP surrounds the many sticky hands of cancer cells, the galectins, keeping them from adhering to one another. This pre-vents the development of cancer clusters and malignant tumors. Cancer cells cannot live alone. They are social cells that need one another. When cancer cells are prevented from attaching to one another, they die.

MCP

Free
Cancer
Cells

**MCP binds to galectin-3
preventing cell interactions**

Cancer Cell Death

MCP Stops the Spread of Cancers

Cancer spreads when malignant cells break away from a primary tumor, travel through the lymph system or bloodstream, and attach themselves to lymph nodes or other organs. These cancer cells can travel great distances. This explains how breast cancer cells may create another tumor on the liver, and how prostate cancer cells can migrate to the lungs. Before clusters of cancer cells can form a secondary tumor, they need to land somewhere, preferably on their food supply—a blood vessel. MCP blocks galectins on the surface of cancer cells, which keeps these clusters from attaching to other sites.

MCP Blocks the Formation of Blood Vessels

Like all living things, cancer cells need food to survive. Blood vessels carry nutrients to all cells. If a tumor attaches itself to an area that has no nearby blood vessels, galectin-3 appears to stimulate the growth of new blood vessels. By destroying galectin-3, MCP keeps new blood vessels from being created and cuts off the cancer cells' food supply.

Degree of Esterification

In addition to its molecular weight, the quality and effectiveness of MCP is determined by its degree of esterification—a way of evaluating its structure. Esterification is a process that makes sugar molecules (galactose) too large for galectins to grab on to. A higher degree of esterification adversely affects pectin's ability to bind to heavy metals, sugar molecules, and other substances. It also keeps galectins from being able to recognize and attach to pectin's sugar molecules.

Think of pectin as being a string of small ball-like sugar molecules and galectins as being hands. The galactose in pectin is just the right size for the hand to grip, like a small ball. Esterification takes that small ball and turns it into a basketball, something that's simply too large for the hand to grip.

The more basketballs (esterified sugar molecules) there are in the pectin chain, the higher the degree of esterification. Ten percent esterification means that every tenth baseball in a pectin chain is a basketball. When a MCP product is made from highly esterified pectin (greater than 50 percent esterification), it contains so many large sugar molecules that the galectins in cancer cells can't even get close enough to the pectin to attach themselves to the chain. If they can't grab on to the pectin, they can attach themselves only to other cancer cells and blood vessels.

This is why you always want a MCP product with a low degree of esterification. Researchers at Wayne State University who have been studying MCP extensively found that the most effective MCP had a starting degree of esterification of 10 percent or less. Part of the research done on MCP by Dr. Eliaz also determined that the optimal esterification was less than 10 percent. Dr. Kenneth Pienta, who conducted the first studies on MCP, agrees with this research. Some of the MCPs that are available have a high degree of esterification—as much as 50 to 70 percent. If the degree of esterification is too high, galectins can't attach themselves to pectin and MCP can't work. Ordinary pectin typically has a degree of esterification of 70 percent.

4. MCP for Prostate Cancer

Of all diseases, MCP has been studied most extensively for prostate cancer. The results of these studies are impressive, and the implications for using MCP for other cancers with the same galectin as prostate cancer, galectin-3, are strong. Before looking into its future applications, we need to look closely at past studies to see just how MCP stops the spread of prostate cancer.

Prostate cancer (PC) is becoming the most common cancer in the world for men, second only to lung cancer. More than 40,000 men in this country alone die of prostate cancer each year. The fact is that most men will get prostate cancer if they live long enough. Statistics show that approximately 70 percent of men over the age of seventy have PC. The good news is that comparatively few will die of it. Still, it is an unpleasant and uncomfortable disease, often interfering with urination, and the majority of men seek treatment for it.

Conventional treatment for prostate cancer includes surgery, radiation, and hormone therapy. Unfortunately, these often result in impotency, incontinence, and loss of libido. Safer treatments are needed and MCP appears to be a strong contender for the first line of defense in preventing prostate cancer and stopping it from spreading to other locations in the body.

Genetics and age are two primary risk factors for PC. But as we learn more about it, we see that PC is not an "old man's disease." While it is more prevalent in men over the age of fifty, young men in their thirties and forties can also get PC. Dr. Stephen Strum is a medical oncologist with a specialty in prostate cancer, as well as the author of an excellent book on the subject, *A Primer on Prostate Can-*

cer (Life Extension Media, 2002). He views prostate cancer and breast cancer as being "brother-sister" diseases and believes there is a hereditary link between the two. Dr. Strum sees a strong similarity between the most effective treatments for both prostate cancer and breast cancer. If you have a family history of either of these cancers, he suggests you get a PSA test at age thirty-five to assess your risk. Otherwise, testing should begin when you reach age forty.

Prostate Cancer Antigen (PSA) Test

There are several screening methods for assessing prostate cancer risk and discovering early PC, but perhaps the one most widely used is the PSA blood test. This test measures the concentration of prostate specific antigen (PSA) in the blood. PSA is an enzyme made by prostate tissue to liquefy semen. The larger the prostate, the more PSA is produced. The presence of cancer raises PSA levels, but other factors raise it as well. They include an enlarged prostate and prostatitis (an inflammatory condition).

Cancer cells in prostate tissues increase the production of PSA ten times faster than normal cells. This is why a baseline PSA test along with a yearly follow-up is so important in helping to identify prostate cancer. Cancer causes PSA to rise more quickly than other factors. Many doctors investigate further for possible prostate cancer if the PSA is greater than 4.0. But Dr. Strum suggests that if your first PSA is 2.0 or higher, it's time for a closer evaluation.

With prostate cancer, tumor cells cause the body to manufacture PSA. The larger the tumor, the more PSA is made. Cancer cells double as they grow and divide: one cell doubles to two, and two cells double to four, and so on. So PSA is measured by looking at the amount of time it takes for the PSA to double. This is called the PSA doubling time (PSADT).

When the PSA doubles in a short period of time, it indicates the possible presence of a malignancy. This PSA doubling time not only helps identify cancer, but also gives an idea of how extensive and aggressive it is. The longer it takes for PSA to double, the slower a tumor is growing—and the less likely it is that prostate cancer is present.

MCP and Prostate Cancer

Unlike conventional treatment for PC, modified citrus pectin is not toxic or invasive. It doesn't result in impotency, loss of libido, bowel problems, or incontinence. MCP has three primary actions: it slows the doubling time of PSA, it stops prostate cancer from spreading, and cancer cell studies show it can kill prostate cancer cells.

MCP Slows PSA Doubling Time

In May 1999, Dr. Strum presented a paper at the International Conference on Diet and Prevention of Cancer in Finland on a small pilot clinical trial using MCP with men who had prostate cancer. This trial found that MCP slowed the PSA doubling time by 50 percent in four out of seven participants. All of the men in this study had either relapsed or failed prior treatment for prostate cancer. Each of them took 15 grams of PectaSol MCP in divided doses for a minimum of six months. In addition to achieving a significant slowing of their PSA doubling time, all men remained alive three years after the study's completion.

The results of this pilot study were confirmed in a small phase II clinical trial headed by Drs. Mark Scholz and Stephen Strum, oncologists with a specialty in prostate cancer, which was presented at the Science of Whole Person Healing Conference (2003). This second study was even more impressive. In it, MCP slowed the doubling time in seven out of ten men with prostate cancer who had low levels of PSA. Once again, each of these men had either relapsed after or failed prior to getting conventional treatment for their prostate cancer. As before, each of the men took 15 grams of PectaSol MCP (six capsules of 800 mg, three times daily), this time for a period of one year. They were encouraged not to make any significant changes to their diets, supplements, or prescription medications so that the investigators could see just what MCP could do. Their PSA doubling time was reduced by more than 50 percent in a full 75 percent of the participants.

MCP Stops the Spread of Prostate Cancer

It is not the primary prostate cancer tumor that is fatal, but the spread of cancer to other locations in the body. Prostate cancer cells can break away from the primary tumor and travel to other sites—often the lungs. When metastasis can be prevented, PC can often be controlled.

Dr. Kenneth Pienta, a pioneer in the field of prostate cancer, conducted an animal study on the oral use of MCP in rats with PC. He found that MCP slowed or stopped its metastasis to the lungs. Fifteen out of sixteen of the control rats in his study developed lung metastases, while at least half of the rats that drank water containing varying amounts of MCP had significantly fewer metastatic colonies.

MCP Kills Prostate Cancer Cells

To further his investigations into the usefulness of MCP for prostate cancer, Dr. Eliaz studied its effect on the adherence of prostate cancer cells to human endothelial tissue cultures. He found that MCP prevented these cancer cells from sticking to endothelial tissue—the tissues that make up blood vessels. MCP didn't just result in the death of a few prostate cancer cells, it prevented 76.9 to 80.7 percent of them from adhering to blood vessel tissues. The results of this study have widespread implications. Blood vessels provide cancer cells with their food supply. Without nourishment, cancer cells die. So by cutting off their source of food, MCP was able to kill prostate cancer cells.

5. MCP for Other Cancers

Cancers of the prostate, breast, colon, lung, brain, kidney, ovaries, and larynx, along with lymphoma, melanoma, leukemia, and glioblastoma, all have galectins (proteins that act like sticky hands) on the surface of their cells—many more galectins than normal cells. Remember that galectins have a particular affinity for sugar molecules, especially galactose—the sugar that's so prevalent in MCP. When galectins attach themselves to MCP molecules, they can't stick to other cancer cells. As long as MCP can get into the bloodstream and its sugar molecules are small enough for the galectins on cancer cells to grab on to, MCP will bind to cancer cells and prevent them from binding to one another. Although there is more research on MCP and prostate cancer, studies strongly support the use of MCP for other cancers as well.

Breast Cancer

Dr. Strum observed a similarity in effective treatments for both prostate cancer and breast cancer. What worked for one, he felt, often worked for another. We've seen in study after study that MCP is effective in fighting prostate cancer, and Dr. Strum's observation is supported by an animal study using MCP on breast cancer, published in the prestigious *Journal of the National Cancer Institute* (2002).

In this study, mice with breast cancer were given varying amounts of MCP in their drinking water. Both doses were effective, but the higher doses of MCP resulted in the greatest reduction in the tumors' growth. It also reduced angiogenesis, which cut off the cancer cells' food supply, and prevented cancer cells from adhering to other sites. Simply stated, this means that MCP reduced breast cancer and prevented breast cancer tumors from forming or spreading.

Colon Cancer

Could modified citrus pectin be effective against colon cancer if most of it is absorbed into the bloodstream? This was a question that needed to be answered, and it was in two studies using laboratory animals by Nangia-Makker and Hayashi. In each study, mice were implanted with colon cancer cells and then given drinking water containing MCP. In each case, there was a significant reduction in the size of the primary tumor, in angiogenesis, and in the spread of cancer to other locations. The results in both of these studies were dose-dependent. The higher doses of MCP resulted in the greatest decreases in tumor size.

These studies are exciting because they were the first ones to show that MCP could reduce the growth of solid primary tumors. Past trials indicated it could stop the spread of cancer (metastasis). These studies found that it could also reduce the size of malignant tumors. If MCP can reduce the size of a tumor that has already taken hold, it can prevent tumors from forming as well.

The manner in which MCP worked was by interfering with galectin-3, the proteins on cancer cells that help them attach to one another. These two studies on colon cancer strongly suggest that MCP will be effective in the prevention and treatment of all types of cancers that contain galectin-3. We may well find through future research that MCP blocks the adhesion of other galectins, as well.

Melanoma

Melanoma is a serious and sometimes fatal form of skin cancer. In fact, in the past thirty years, the number of cases of melanoma in this country has doubled. The greatest danger with melanoma is when melanoma cells migrate through the skin and attach themselves to a secondary site, such as another organ. Can MCP prevent melanoma from spreading? Let's take a look at two studies comparing citrus pectin with modified citrus pectin on melanoma cells and in animals that were injected with melanoma cells.

The first study conducted by Platt and Raz, and published in the *Journal of the National Cancer Institute,* showed that when melanoma cells were exposed to ordinary citrus pectin, tumor colonies increased up to three times. In other words, ordinary pectin had no blocking effect. But when MCP was injected, metastasis decreased by 90 percent!

These results were duplicated in a second test-tube study by Inohara and Raz. In this study, MCP prevented the melanoma cells from adhering to tissues. The authors suggest that the reason for this is the attraction for galectin-3 in lung cancer cells to the sugar molecules in MCP. This, they think, is what keeps melanoma cells from traveling to other sites, attaching themselves to other organs, and spreading.

6. MCP Prevents Cancer

How is it possible to say that MCP prevents cancer? Quite simply, Dr. Pienta's animal study showed that modified citrus pectin prevented prostate cancer cells from attaching themselves to blood vessels. In the control group, cancer cells migrated to the lungs and colonized, forming secondary malignant tumors. In more than half of the other groups, cancer cells simply couldn't take hold. MCP appears to have strong anti-angiogenesis properties.

When cancer is developing, it is less aggressive than when it has grown into a malignant tumor. Individual cancer cells have fewer galectins to bind to other cells, so its colonies grow more slowly. As cancer progresses, its cells get more galectins that grab onto one another and to blood vessels more readily. This is why a slow growing cancer needs much less MCP to interfere with the formation of tumors than an advanced cancer.

Based on the dramatic results of his clinical trial on the slowing down of PSA doubling time, along with all of the other studies that have been conducted with MCP, Dr. Eliaz is now using modified citrus pectin as a major nutraceutical in his clinic for the prevention of cancer. While he believes that 3 to 5 grams a day may be sufficient, Dr. Eliaz begins by giving his patients the full 15 gram-per-day dose for one month. He uses this high dose in order to have "a scavenger effect". For one month, he lets MCP aggressively seek and destroy any cancer cells.

7. The Future of MCP

We've just begun to scratch the surface of all that MCP can do, but the studies that have already been conducted give us a preview of what we expect to find as research into this important substance progresses. There has been a great deal of research conducted on ordinary pectin, a fiber with molecules too large to get into the bloodstream. Whatever pectin can do in the intestinal tract appears to be what modified citrus pectin can do when it can be absorbed into the bloodstream and make its way into tissues throughout the body.

This has serious implications for MCP's many benefits in the area of heart disease and immunity. But its value doesn't stop with these diseases. As science searches for the causes of age-related illnesses, we have reason to believe that MCP may be able to stop and even reverse Alzheimer's disease. The enhanced capabilities of modified citrus pectin over ordinary citrus pectin are enabling researchers to look in a number of different directions to find out just how much this nutraceutical can do. Here are some of the most promising applications on the horizon for MCP:

Lowering Cholesterol

We know from numerous studies that soluble fiber, the type found in ordinary pectin, binds to cholesterol in the gut and lowers total cholesterol levels. It also lowers LDL, the sticky cholesterol that leads to a buildup of plaque and heart disease.

In a double-blind, placebo-controlled trial headed by Dr. James Cerda and published in *Clinical Cardiology* in 1988, participants who

were at a medium-to-high risk for heart disease and had high cholesterol levels were given a pectin supplement over a period of four
months. They made no other changes in their daily routine. Their
diets remained the same and their exercising—or lack of exercising—
weren't altered. The results of this study were encouraging. Pectin
alone reduced their total cholesterol by 7.6 percent and lowered their
LDL ("harmful") cholesterol by more than 10 percent. This study
concluded that adding citrus pectin to the diet can significantly
reduce cholesterol.

At first glance this seems impressive. That is, until you start reading studies on the actions of modified citrus pectin. Because MCP
binds to cholesterol in the bloodstream as well as in the intestines, its
effectiveness in reducing cholesterol in the blood and liver should far
exceed that of ordinary pectin. However, we don't have studies at this
time on MCP and cholesterol.

The role of cholesterol in heart disease is under scrutiny. The lat-
est information suggests that it is not just any form of cholesterol that
is harmful, but an oxidized cholesterol called oxysterol. Oxysterols are
formed from exposure to environmental pollutants. When they get
into the bloodstream, they can cause a buildup of plaque to be
formed in arteries, leading to atherosclerosis. Before you can reduce
atherosclerosis, you need to reduce toxins in the blood and tissues.

Reducing Atherosclerosis

A high level of oxidized cholesterol puts you at a greater risk for heart
disease because it can lead to atherosclerosis. In atherosclerosis, the
walls of the arteries to the brain and heart become harder and thicker
from deposits of plaque often resulting in angina, heart attacks, or
stroke. Pectin has other binding abilities that are not yet completely
understood that reduce atherosclerosis.

In a nine-month study of animals with high cholesterol, 3 percent of the cellulose in their diet was exchanged for 3 percent grapefruit pectin. Interestingly, there was no significant change in total
cholesterol levels. There was, however, a greater reduction of plaque
in the aortas and coronary arteries in those animals that were given
pectin than in the control group that ate a diet higher in cellulose.

This study was conducted using ordinary pectin. We expect that MCP will be even more effective against atherosclerosis because of its ability to bind to excessive calcium in arteries, to heavy metals, and to environmental pollutants.

Removing Environmental Toxins

In the early 1990s, after the accident at the Chernobyl atomic electric power station, scientists rushed to find a way to remove radiation metabolites from the many thousands of people who had been exposed. Some of these scientists thought to use pectin because of its superior binding capacities, and pectin worked beautifully. Incidents of radiation sickness declined dramatically. In study after study, pectin removed toxic substances like plutonium and strontium from the intestines of Russians exposed to radiation. By removing toxins in the gut, MCP prevented some of these toxic substances from entering the bloodstream and becoming trapped in tissues.

Dr. Sherry A. Rogers is a medical doctor who has written a number of well-documented books on the relationship between toxicity and disease, including *Tired or Toxic?* (Prestige Publishing, 1990). She has seen the connection between toxins and chronic illnesses in her patients for decades. Dr. Rogers has found that foreign chemicals, called xenobiotics, are a major contributing factor to illnesses that range from depression to chronic fatigue and a lowered immune system. Only through effective detoxification, she finds, can health be restored in the majority of her severely ill patients.

Ordinary pectin may be sufficient for someone who suffers from a single acute toxic exposure to a contaminant, but most people have been exposed to low levels of a variety of pollutants over a period of years. For them, ordinary pectin would do little to lower their toxic load. Only MCP can enter the bloodstream and remove toxins from the blood and tissues. As researchers look to pesticides and other environmental pollutants as being an underlying cause of chronic illnesses, the use of MCP in health care will expand.

Removing Heavy Metals

Heavy metals are everywhere. From cadmium in cigarette smoke, mercury in fish and dental fillings, and lead in pesticides and paints, heavy metals permeate our air, water, and food supply. At one time, Dr. Rogers was alone in her association between toxins and disease. Now, more than ever, doctors of complementary medicine are pointing to heavy metal toxicity as being a major underlying cause of a variety of degenerative illnesses. We may be able to reduce using so many toxic substances in the future, but there's no way to eliminate heavy metals from our environment. What we can do, however, is to keep eliminating them from our bodies.

Heavy metals have been implicated in a wide number of health problems, including arteriosclerosis, hypertension, multiple sclerosis, impaired immune function, and an overgrowth of *Candida albicans*. Women with persistent cases of *Candida albicans* who have tried everything else may have high levels of mercury. If so, modified citrus pectin will bind to mercury both in the bowel and in the bloodstream, and slowly help eliminate it.

Research exists showing the effectiveness of pectin in chelating (binding to) heavy metals and removing them from the body. In one study, 3–4 grams of a pectin preparation were given to a group of workers with an occupational exposure to lead. They took the pectin for a month and had an increased excretion of lead. The authors suggest that people who have a continued exposure to lead should take regular courses of pectin to reduce their toxic load. By using modified citrus pectin instead, it should be possible to reduce contaminants in the blood and tissues as well as in the intestines.

Although there are few studies using MCP for heavy metals, a Russian study compared pectins with varying degrees of esterification (the process that affects the size of its sugar molecules). The pectin with the lowest degree of esterification blocked the absorption of lead the best. If you'll remember, pectin with a low degree of esterification has more small sugar molecules. This strongly suggests that MCP with a low degree of esterification could best bind to heavy metals in the bloodstream and tissues.

Time, and research, will tell. A pilot trial is now underway that will combine modified alginate from seaweed with PectaSol MCP. Each substance chelates different amounts of various heavy metals in the gut and bloodstream, and each has different binding properties. Modified alginate binds better to mercury and modified citrus pectin binds better to lead. By combining the two and looking for the optimal balance of ingredients, researchers hope to find a product specifically targeted to remove a wide number of heavy metals. Human clinical trials will follow this pilot study and results are expected in a few years.

Preventing and Reducing Alzheimer's Disease

Scientists are constantly uncovering new applications for modified citrus pectin, and occasionally an idea will come seemingly out of nowhere. Along with its many known uses, MCP may turn out to be an important substance for the prevention and treatment of Alzheimer's disease. A recent article, published in the respected medical journal *The Lancet* (February 15, 2003), suggests this may be so. We know that MCP is anti-angiogenic, and current thought now under investigation points to a direct connection between angiogenesis (the formation of new blood vessels) and Alzheimer's disease.

The rationale for using MCP for Alzheimer's disease began with the observation that particular medications appear to reduce a person's risk for dementia. One theory is that Alzheimer's disease is caused, at least in part, by an inflammation in the brain's blood vessels. Could inflammation in the brain—a focus of current research—be the reason these drugs worked? Probably not, since not all of the anti-Alzheimer's drugs had anti-inflammatory activity. What each of the drugs studied had in common, however, were anti-angiogenic properties.

This article in *The Lancet,* written by Drs. Vagnucci, Jr. and Li, of Cambridge, Massachusetts, suggests that inflammation is just one trigger for the production of new blood vessels, and that it is this new blood vessel growth that causes the deposit of plaque and the secretion of a toxin that kills brain cells, leading to Alzheimer's disease. This toxin is secreted by blood vessels in all of us as we age, but the brains of people with Alzheimer's disease secrete much larger quantities than those of people without dementia. If angiogenesis can be stopped, these doctors theorize, so can the progression of Alzheimer's disease.

Discussion is underway between a doctor who has conducted research on MCP and the authors of this article. The next step is to begin laboratory and clinical studies. If MCP can stop, or even slow down, the progression of Alzheimer's disease–related angiogenesis, it may be possible to successfully treat or prevent this disease. If preliminary studies suggest it can, this will place MCP high on the list of anti-aging supplements.

8. How to Use MCP

Ordinary pectin is limited to traveling within the digestive tract. Just like all fibers, large amounts can cause loose stools and gas. MCP, on the other hand, travels in the bloodstream as well as in the intestines, so some of it will be eliminated through solid wastes, and some in the urine. This reduces incidents of digestive disturbances.

At its full dose, MCP only causes mild flatulence and loose stools 5 percent of the time. If you experience either of these symptoms, reduce your dosage and slowly increase it until you reach the suggested levels.

Suggested Dosage

The suggested dosages are based on those from studies conducted on MCP. The optimal dose for slowing metastasis is around 15 grams a day. Before and after surgeries or biopsies where cancer is suspected, begin by taking 15 grams of MCP a day for one week before the procedure. Continue taking this amount for two to four weeks afterward, depending on the size of the procedure. In other words, the more complicated the surgery, the longer the optimal dose of MCP should be taken.

With cancer therapy, MCP may be used after chemotherapy ends or during the week before commencement of chemotherapy in a three-week cycle. It may be used along with radiation therapy unless your digestive system is too sensitive. In these cases, take 5–15 grams a day—the highest amount that can be taken without discomfort. Some individuals with metastatic disease may find that when 15 grams per day is not sufficient, a higher dosage of 20–25 grams may produce results. Although this is not a recommended dose based on studies, MCP is nontoxic, and a higher dose is worth trying for anyone with an advanced disease who doesn't respond to 15 grams.

For cancer prevention, 3–5 grams a day may be sufficient, but higher doses are not a problem since the density of galectin-3 molecules increases as the disease progresses.

- MCP should be taken in three equally divided amounts.
- For serious existing conditions: 15 grams daily.
- For preventive measures: Begin with 15 grams daily for one month, then 3–5 grams daily thereafter.
- For long-term exposure to toxins: 3–5 grams daily.

How Long Should You Take MCP?

MCP works as long as it is in your bloodstream and comes into contact with certain substances. You should use it for as long as it takes to reduce your toxic load, remove arterial plaque, prevent blood vessel formation, or block cancer cells from attaching to one another or to arteries.

The more serious your condition, the longer you should use the optimal dose of 15 grams daily as determined through animal studies, *in vitro* studies, and human clinical trials. People with active cancer should continue using 15 grams of MCP a day on a permanent basis.

If budget is an issue, a cancer patient in remission could, after two to three years, reduce their dosage to 5–10 grams a day. Some people will want to use a lower dose as part of their permanent daily supplementation to prevent cancer, heart disease, and other conditions.

9. Choosing MCP Products

The quality of available MCP products varies widely. Some actually contain no modified citrus pectin as it's been defined here. "Modified" means "changed," and there are supplement companies that are selling ordinary, large-molecule citrus pectin with additional nutrients like vitamin C and soy protein under the name of Modified Citrus Protein. This is unfortunate, because while it may be legal to do this, people with cancer, heart disease, or heavy metal toxicity who use ordinary pectin products cannot possibly get the results they're seeking—the results suggested from solid research.

Before you buy any brand of MPC, read the label carefully. Has the pectin actually been modified to reduce the size of its molecules, or is someone just misleading you? Begin by avoiding any products that do not list modified citrus pectin in the ingredients list.

Next, you may want to contact the manufacturer of an MCP product to find out its molecular weight and degree of esterification, since there are no requirements that these be listed on the label.

Choose Quality Over Price

The enzymatic process used to modify the highest-quality pectin is expensive. Lower-priced products are not produced with this process. Don't expect to get the same results with an inexpensive brand that you'll get from one that costs more. This is one instance where you don't want to shop around for the least expensive product. This said, your choice remains between a MCP product that has been tested in research studies and one that has not.

The molecular weight and degree of esterification varies greatly between MCP products. The only studies to date have been done on MCPs with a molecular weight of between 10,000 and 20,000 daltons and with ten degrees of esterification or less. You can call a manufacturer and ask about the weight and structure of their product, or you can choose the only product that has been clinically tested—PectaSol. If you use a brand that hasn't been tested and don't get the results you expect, you may want to try PectaSol.

Based on clinical studies, to be effective against cancer and heart disease a modified citrus pectin product should have:

• A molecular weight of between 10,000 and 20,000 daltons

• 10 percent (or less) degree of esterification

Presently, MCP is sold solely as a nutritional supplement, but its use is expected to expand in time. Researchers at Wayne State University are working hard to develop a MCP molecule for the pharmaceutical industry to be given intravenously. This will allow it to get directly into the bloodstream where, due to their molecular size and structure, some oral forms may not. When it has been developed, this drug will be much more expensive than any form of oral MCP.

If a modified citrus pectin product is of the proper molecular size and degree of esterification, it should not be necessary to use intravenous MCP. If, on the other hand, the size and structure of a particular MCP product doesn't permit it to be fully absorbed and utilized, the drug would be useful.

Because of its safety and wide applications, an oral modified citrus pectin product that can get into the bloodstream and bind to undesirable substances should always be available.

10. Auxiliary Products

MCP is meant to be used as a vital part of an integrated dietary and supplement program. Always begin your program with a good quality multivitamin/mineral and add other specific nutrients according to your condition.

For example, in cases of cancer and other conditions where immune deficiency exists, MCP may be combined with such immune enhancers as medicinal mushroom compounds and thymus gland products. Prostate cancer patients will want to include a supplement containing saw palmetto, nettles, and pygeum, and breast cancer patients will want to add nutrients such as indole-3- carbinol and calcium d-glucarate. When the digestive tract has been damaged, whether through heavy metals or the use of antibiotics, probiotics should be added for a period of three to six months to help restore the balance of friendly bacteria.

While MCP binds to undesirable substances and removes them from the body, other nutrients accelerate the healing process. MCP has been tested as a single substance, but it may work even better when combined with other supplements according to individual need.

Conclusion

We are poised at the beginning of a new age: the Age of Nutraceuticals. Historically, we have seen that plants hold the secrets to many of our health problems and that pharmaceutical companies do not have the only effective products. The manufacturers of nutritional supplements are working today along parallel lines to conduct studies on plant derivatives that are more closely related to plants than their synthetic cousins.

These plant products and their components hold promises of greater health and a longer life at a fraction of the cost of pharmaceuticals. Modified citrus pectin is rapidly being recognized as one of the most important single nutraceuticals available today for both the prevention and treatment of serious illnesses. Scientific studies have demonstrated its usefulness in a number of different kinds of cancers, and its implications for heart disease and for removing heavy metal toxicity are both obvious and exciting. The studies that are being planned, or are underway, are expected to elicit still more applications.

These scientific studies are extremely important in evaluating any product. Without them, we can't know either their effectiveness or their limitations. Anything can be said about a product—and often is. New "natural" products with lofty claims are appearing on the market almost daily. Many of these claims are based on folklore and instinct. Without solid research, we just can't know whether or not they're valid. Other products, not identical to those being studied, are riding on the coattails of science. Such is the case with MCP.

What we know about this product is from studies using modified citrus pectin of a particular molecular weight and with a specific structure. The size of MCP's molecules is critical to its ability to get into the bloodstream and survive. Its structure determines whether or not it can bind to cancer cells or heavy metals, and if so, how well. Until MCPs with different molecular weights and structures are studied, no one knows what they can do.

At a time when doctors are using more and more drugs, all with side effects, we need nontoxic substances like never before. But even more important, we need natural products that have been thoroughly studied in clinical trials that medical doctors can feel comfortable integrating into their protocols. Modified citrus pectin is one of them. Now that you have seen what MCP can do, you may want to share this booklet with your doctor. Together, you can determine your next step in the prevention or treatment of a number of diseases.

Resources

PectaSol® (the only modified citrus pectin product that has been clinically tested) is manufactured exclusively for and is distributed by:

> **EcoNugenics, Inc.**
> *Provides free technical support.*
> (800) 308-5518
> www.econugenics.com

PectaSol is also available from the following distributors:

Longevity Science	**Pure Encapsulations**
(800) 993-9440	(800) 753-2277
www.longevity-science.net	www.purecaps.com
Douglas Laboratories	**Professional Health Products**
(888) 368-4522 (In U.S.)	(403) 227-3926 (In U.S.)
(866) 856-9954 (In Canada)	(800) 661-1366 (In Canada)
www.douglaslabs.com	www.professionalhealthproducts.com

Untested modified citrus pectin products are available from the following distributors, who may also carry PectaSol:

Jarrow Formulas	**Source Naturals**
(800) 726-0886	Customer service: (800) 815-2333
Call for store locations.	

For More Information on Prostate Cancer:

Stephen Strum, M.D., and Donna Pogliano. *A Primer on Prostate Cancer: The Empowered Patient's Guide.* Hollywood, FL: Life Extension Foundation, 2002.

Better Health Publishing at www.dreliaz.com

References

Baekey PA, Cerda JJ, et al., "Grapefruit pectin inhibits hypercholesterolemia and atherosclerosis in miniature swine," *Clin Cardiol,* 1988: 11(9):597–600.

Bereza, Vla, et al., "Pectin-containing products in the dietary nutrition of subjects exposed to ionizing radiation as a result of the accident at the Chernobyl Atomic Electric Power Station," *Lik Sprava,* 1993 Jul; (8):21–4.

Bondarev, GI, et al., "Evaluation of a pectin with a low degree of esterification as a prophylactic agent in lead poisoning," *Vopr Pitan,* 1979, Mar–Apr; (2):65-7.

Cerda, JJ, et al., "The effects of grapefruit pectin on patients at risk for coronary heart disease without altering diet or lifestyle," *Clin Cardiol,* 1988: 11:589–594.

Frankel, Stephen, et al., "Screening for prostate cancer," *The Lancet,* March 29, 2003.

Goldberg, Burton, *Alternative Medicine: The Definitive Guide,* Second Edition, Alternative Medicine.com, 2002.

Guess, Brad, Scholz, Mark, Strum, Stephen, et al., "Modified Citrus Pectin (MCP) increases the prostate specific antigen doubling time in men with prostate cancer: A Phase II clinical trial," paper presented at the Science of Whole Person Healing Conference, 2003, Washington, D.C. Paper available from EcoNugenics.

Hayashi, A, et al., "Effects of daily oral administration of quercetin chalcone and modified citrus pectin on implanted colon-25 tumor growth in balb-c mice," *Alternative Medicine Review,* 2000; (5)6.

Hendler, Sheldon Saul, Ph.D., M.D., and Rorvik, David, MS, PDR for Nutritional Supplements, Medical Economics Company, Inc, Montvale, NJ, 2001.

Hexeberg, E, et al., "A study on lipid metabolism in heart and liver of cholesterol- and pectin-fed rats," *Br J Nutr,* 1994, Feb, 71(2):181-92.

Inohara, H and Raz, A, "Effects of natural complex carbohydrate (citrus pectin) on murine melanoma cell properties related to galectin-3 functions," *Glycoconj J,* 1994; 11(6): 527–32.

Moss, Ralph W, Ph.D., Cancer Therapy, Equinox Press, Brooklyn, NY, 1997.

Nangia-Makker, Pratima, et al., "Inhibition of human cancer cell growth and metastasis in nude mice by oral intake of modified citrus pectin," *J Natl Cancer Inst,* 2002; 94:1854-62.

Pienta, KJ, et al., "Inhibition of spontaneous metastatis in a rat prostate cancer model by oral administration of modified citrus pectin," *J Natl Cancer Inst,* March 1, 1995, 1:87(5):348–53.

Platt, D and Raz, A, "Modulation of the lung colonization of B16-F1 melanoma cells by citrus pectin," *J Natl Cancer Inst,* 1994; 84(6):438–42.

Rogers, Sherry A, M.D., *Tired or Toxic?,* Prestige Publishing, 1990.

Romanenko, AE, et al., "Further improvement in the administration of pectin as a preventive agent against absorption of radionuclides by human body," *Gig Tr Prof Zabol,* 1991;(12):8–10.

Strum, Stephen B, M.D. and Pogliano, Donna, *A Primer on Prostate Cancer,* Life Extension Media, Hollywood, FL, 2002.

Taylor, Norman, *Plant Drugs That Changed the World,* Dodd, Mead & Company, 1965.

Trakhtenberg, IM, et al., "The prophylactic use of pectin in chronic lead exposure," *Lik Sprava,* 1995, Jan-Feb (1–2):132–6.

Vagnucci Jr,, Anthony H and Li, William W, "Alzheimer's disease and angiogenesis," *The Lancet,* Feb 15, 2003 (wli@angio.org).

Watanabe, K, et al., "Effect of dietary alfalfa, pectin, and wheat bran on azoxymethane- or methylnitrosourea-induced colon carcinogenesis in F344 rats," *J Natl Cancer Inst,* 1979; 63:141–5.

Weiss, Tania, Ph.D., "Modified Citrus Pectin" induces cytotoxicity of prostate cancer cells in co-cultures with human endothelial monolayers," paper presented at the International Conference on Diet and Prevention of Cancer, May 1999, Tampere, Finland.

Index

About the Author

Nan Kathryn Fuchs, Ph.D., is a nutritionist in private practice in Sebastopol, California, as well as a health educator. She is author of several books, including *The Nutrition Detective, Overcoming the Legacy of Overeating,* and *The Giant Book of Women's Health Secrets.* She is also nutrition editor for the *Women's Health Letter,* a popular newsletter.

The BASIC HEALTH GUIDE Series

Basic Health Guides are informational booklets published regularly to provide you with the newest and best available data on health subjects of major importance. Basic Health Guides are written by leading physicians, doctors, pharmacists, and nutrition-oriented reporters.

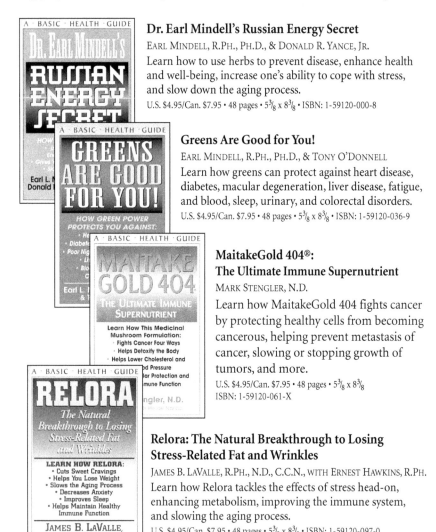

Dr. Earl Mindell's Russian Energy Secret

EARL MINDELL, R.PH., PH.D., & DONALD R. YANCE, JR.

Learn how to use herbs to prevent disease, enhance health and well-being, increase one's ability to cope with stress, and slow down the aging process.

U.S. $4.95/Can. $7.95 • 48 pages • $5^3/_8$ x $8^3/_8$ • ISBN: 1-59120-000-8

Greens Are Good for You!

EARL MINDELL, R.PH., PH.D., & TONY O'DONNELL

Learn how greens can protect against heart disease, diabetes, macular degeneration, liver disease, fatigue, and blood, sleep, urinary, and colorectal disorders.

U.S. $4.95/Can. $7.95 • 48 pages • $5^3/_8$ x $8^3/_8$ • ISBN: 1-59120-036-9

MaitakeGold 404®: The Ultimate Immune Supernutrient

MARK STENGLER, N.D.

Learn how MaitakeGold 404 fights cancer by protecting healthy cells from becoming cancerous, helping prevent metastasis of cancer, slowing or stopping growth of tumors, and more.

U.S. $4.95/Can. $7.95 • 48 pages • $5^3/_8$ x $8^3/_8$
ISBN: 1-59120-061-X

Relora: The Natural Breakthrough to Losing Stress-Related Fat and Wrinkles

JAMES B. LAVALLE, R.PH., N.D., C.C.N., WITH ERNEST HAWKINS, R.PH.

Learn how Relora tackles the effects of stress head-on, enhancing metabolism, improving the immune system, and slowing the aging process.

U.S. $4.95/Can. $7.95 • 48 pages • $5^3/_8$ x $8^3/_8$ • ISBN: 1-59120-097-0

.

Printed in the USA
CPSIA information can be obtained
at www.ICGtesting.com
JSHW012010140824
68134JS00004B/102

9 781681 626772